Incredible Herbal Remedies!

Herbal Remedies

Herbs, Spices, And Oils To Cure Common Ailments, Prevent Sickness, Improve Health And Fight Disease!

I0420138

Sarah Brooks

STOP!!! Before you read any further....Would you like to know the secrets of Anti Aging?

If your answer is yes, then you are not alone. Thousands of people are looking for the secret to reducing wrinkles, looking younger, and maintaining a youthful appearance.

If you have been searching for these answers without much luck, you are in the right place!

Not only will you gain incredible insight in this book, but because I want to make sure to give you as much value as possible, right now for a limited time you can get full **100% FREE access to a VIP bonus Ebook** entitled **Anti Aging Made Easy!**

Just Go Here For Free Instant Access:

www.LuxyLifeNaturals.com

Legal Notice

Disclaimer Notice

the author and publisher reserve the right to alter and update the information contained herein on the new conditions whenever they see applicable.

Table of Contents

Introduction

I want to thank you and congratulate you for purchasing the book, *"Herbal Remedies: Incredible Herbal Remedies! - Herbs, Spices, And Oils To Cure Common Ailments, Prevent Sickness, Improve Health And Fight Disease!"*

This "Herbal Remedies" book contains proven steps and strategies on how to:

- Benefit from affordable, safer and effective treatments for common ailments, chronic conditions and diseases using herbal remedies;

- Prevent sickness with herbs, spices and essential oils;

- Use the healing powers of herbs, spices and oils to improve your health;

- Do oil pulling to stop and prevent tooth decay, gum problems and improve your oral health;

- Use herbs as your natural anti-aging solution so you don't have to spend much for costly skin care products;

- Use honey for medicinal purposes;

- Use apple cider vinegar for weight loss;

- Start sustainable gardening of herbal plants.

These and more are yours to enjoy when you start reading the contents of this book. Use this book as your guide to benefit from one of Mother Nature's greatest gifts to humanity - incredible herbal remedies.

Why entrust your life entirely on pharmaceutical medicines when you can benefit from herbal remedies for health conditions that do not necessitate medical intervention?

Thanks again for purchasing this book. I hope you enjoy it!

Chapter 1: 4 Incredible Things Herbal Remedies Can Do

Herbal remedies continue to increase in popularity. More and more people choose to benefit from these natural remedies to treat their ailments and protect their health. In fact, the World Health Organization (WHO) approximates that about 80% of the entire world population include herbal medicines as part of their health treatment.

In this chapter, you will discover four (4) of the incredible things that herbal remedies can do. You may have not yet known about some of these things and your physician may never tell you about the other things.

More Affordable Treatment

Using herbs as natural remedies enables you to save your hard-earned money. Saving money may not be possible with pharmaceutical medicines given their typically high cost. Aside from being the more affordable solution for ailments, botanical remedies are also equally effective compared to drug-based medications.

The Harvard Medical School recognizes the ability of botanicals to heal. In fact, it has published a special health report on how to treat common pain conditions without using drugs or surgery. Results from several studies and research likewise show that plant-based medications work well with the body systems.

Safer Treatment than Drugs

Herbs and other natural remedies are safer treatment than drug-based medicines. Typically, herbal medicines do not carry side effects because of their natural composition. Drugs, on the other hand, contain active ingredients that interfere with the body systems; hence, the side effects.

Side effects of pharmaceutical medicines often occur (a) when you start taking the medication, (b) change the dosage either to lower it or to strengthen it and (c) when you stop taking your medicine(s). In contrast, the side effects that may happen with herbal treatments are normally attributable to the improper use of the medication.

Potency Similar to Pharmaceuticals

At first glance, herbal medicines may not be as potent as pharmaceutical medicines when it comes to comparing their dosage. For instance, a cup of tea of willow bark (naturally containing aspirin and works as a pain reliever) is weaker in dosage than the standard dosage of pharmaceutical aspirin.

However, instead of looking at the dosage comparison, look at the effects of these medications. If taking a cup of willow bark can suffice to relieve your pain, why risk your general health to the typical side effects of pharmaceutical medicines? Keep in mind a general rule in medication: start taking your medicine with the lowest dosage possible.

More Effective Treatment for Chronic Conditions

Unless your medical condition needs urgent intervention or treatment, herbal remedies are usually more effective than drug-based medications. With chronic conditions, treatment may require a longer period involving repeated use of the medication(s). This could mean greater risks of side effects with pharmaceuticals.

Botanicals, on the other hand, have no side effects or minimal side effects only. As mentioned earlier, the side effects typically occur only with improper use or dosage. Herbs contain natural chemicals that can sufficiently address chronic health conditions without the risk of side effects.

Chapter 2: Prevent Sickness With Natural Remedies

If drug-based medicines are most beneficial during emergencies, you would enjoy the maximum benefits of natural remedies if you use them to prevent diseases. In this chapter, you'll discover the power of the botanicals as natural solutions in preventing sickness.

Origin

The power of plants to heal, treat and cure sickness has its root from ancient medical practice. Ancient physicians did not only use plants to treat diseases, but also they studied the healing properties of these plants to gather materials for creating standards and treatises.

Even modern medicines have their roots on botanicals. In fact, most of the pharmaceuticals today contain active ingredients from plants. What drug companies do is they isolate the chemicals found in botanicals and use them as active ingredients. This way, they can patent the formula, which is not possible with whole herbs.

Scientific Proof

Perhaps due to the unstoppable growth in the popularity of botanicals as natural remedies, more studies now provide the scientific proof for the healing powers of herbs and other plants.

However, you may want to know why herbs do not get as much evidence despite the number of people who have attested the effectiveness of the natural remedies. Here are the reasons:

- Lack of Funds – Scientific and clinical tests and trials are costly. It is rare that a company will fund these tests if they do not foresee any returns on their investment. In other words, since herbs are not patentable, companies cannot profit from them; hence, they seldom fund such tests.

- No Patent – There is no way to secure a patent for whole herbs. This is the reason why drug companies usually "purify" the chemicals and use them in their "purified" form as active ingredients, so they can patent for higher profitability. Drug companies are the ones that normally support and fund studies and research.

- Difficult Format for Testing – Pharmaceuticals make it difficult for herbs to follow the prescribed format for testing and measuring how they work in the body. Typically, how herbs work depend on the unique condition of the individual, unlike drug-based medicines where there is a standard formulation and dosage requirement.

Chapter 3: Herbs, Spices, And Oils To Cure Common Ailments And To Improve Health

Do you know that in your home is where you will find perhaps the best solutions to improve health and cure common ailments? In this chapter, you'll discover the healing properties of herbs, spices and oils.

3 Herbs that Heal

Here are three (3) of the best herbs that cure common ailments:

1. Ginger – You can easily stop and prevent nausea and stomach upset with ginger. If you wish to prevent airsickness, take ginger before you board the plane or at least 30 minutes before takeoff.

   Ginger improves your health by regulating your blood pressure, lowering your risks of cancer, as well as preventing and relieving your pain from osteoarthritis. Most people also find ginger effective for sore throat.

2. Holy Basil – which is popular among pesto lovers can be your anti-stress and anxiety medication. The plant regulates your stress hormone and improves the response mechanism of your body to stress and anxiety.

   Rich in antioxidants, the holy basil can treat multiple common ailments such as but not limited to common colds, digestive problems, ulcers and bronchitis. It also enhances the immune system to increase the body's natural defense against infections and diseases.

3. Sage – is an effective natural remedy for headaches, sinusitis, sores, respiratory ailments, and fever. You can also apply sage solution topically to treat skin itchiness, scalp problems and wounds.

You can also use sage as a disinfectant because of its antimicrobial properties. It can also improve your focus and your memory. However, refrain from using sage if you are pregnant or nursing your infant. Long-term use must have the approval of your herbalist.

3 Spices that Soothe your Stomach

The most common ailments usually occur or start with stomach disorders. Here are three (3) of the best spices that can soothe stomach health problems.

4. Black Pepper – is a popular natural remedy for intestinal gas. It is also effective for treating indigestion and diarrhea.

   This spice can help improve your general health by preventing obesity and skin diseases. Its anti-parasitic properties make it an effective solution to get rid of intestinal parasites.

5. Cinnamon – treats common digestive disorders, such as but not limited to reflux, ulcers, constipation and diarrhea, hemorrhoids, vomiting and stomach pain. It can prevent urinary tract infection and lower your high blood pressure specifically triglycerides.

6. Parsley – is another popular remedy for stomach upset. As one of the most effective healing spices, it can treat and prevent multiple health conditions naturally. Some of these conditions are the following: anemia, gout, bad breath, diarrhea, digestive problems, gallstones, kidney problems and liver congestion.

2 Essential Oils that Energize

Your body needs energy to do its normal functions as well as to increase physical activity necessary to maintain good health. Lack of energy is often a signal of probable health issues. Here are two (2) essential oils that can energize:

7. Citrus oil – helps clear your body of toxins. These toxins interfere with your body systems, making you feel lethargic. It also improves the functions of your lymphatic system to protect your heart health and boost your immune system.

8. Peppermint oil- is a natural energy booster. Aside from increasing your energy, this oil can also improve your satiety that is important in managing your weight. Most people also use peppermint to soothe stomach pain and other digestive problems.

Chapter 4: Fight Disease With Super Herbs And Spices

You don't have to spend much to fight disease. You can win the battles and even the war using herbs and spices as your artillery. In this chapter, you'll learn what herbs and spices to use to win the war against top five chronic conditions.

Heart Disease

Heart attack and stroke are two of the most common life threatening cardiovascular diseases. Risk factors are the following: high blood pressure, high cholesterol, obesity or excess weight, diabetes, sedentary lifestyle, genetics and age (50 years above).

Herbs and spices can prevent heart disease and most of its risk factors. Here are two of the best herbs and spices that promote heart health:

1. Garlic – Since the ancient times, garlic has been a popular anti-inflammatory and antibacterial agent. The father of medicine, Hippocrates, recommended garlic as a part of the treatment for infection, digestive problems, leprosy, cancer and wounds.

   Modern medicine acknowledges the healing powers of garlic. Cardiologists would even include it in their prescription for promoting cardiovascular health.

2. Cilantro – is rich in beta-carotene, an antioxidant that promotes heart health. This herb can lower your risks of heart attacks and stroke. It can remove toxins from your body, most especially mercury (which you can get from food, dental fillings and exposure to some household products).

Diabetics will benefit much from cilantro. Aside from protecting the condition of your heart, this herb can regulate the production of toxic metabolites.

Cancer

You can prevent cancer with the help of super herbs and spices, such as the following:

3. Turmeric – contains <u>curcumin</u>, a powerful natural chemical that fights and prevents inflammation. Curcumin chokes cancer cells until they die. Regular intake of turmeric can prevent cancer cells from forming in the body.

4. Oregano – has <u>carvacrol</u>, a natural chemical that gives oregano its warm odor and can also inhibit the formation of cancer cells in the body. It also protects the body against infections and reduces <u>HCA (heterocyclic amine)</u>, a substance that can trigger cancer growth.

Type 2 Diabetes

As part of the natural treatment for Type 2 diabetes, these herbs can regulate your blood sugar levels:

5. Bitter Melon – It can lower your high blood sugar. What this plant does in the body is that it boosts the ability of the cells to use blood sugar effectively. It also contains antioxidants that protect the body from the harmful effects of unregulated blood sugar.

6. Onions – Along with raw garlic, raw onions can reduce the levels of glucose (blood sugar) and increase insulin in individuals who already have Type 2 diabetes. Onions do not reduce blood sugar levels of healthy individuals.

Chapter 5: 5 Essential Oils With Incredible Health Benefits

Essential oils are popular for aromatherapy. However, there are many other uses of these oils such as: (a) topical solution; (b) massage therapy; (c) bathwater solution to name some. These oils can improve your physical, mental and emotional health. In this chapter, you will discover five (5) essential oils with incredible health benefits.

Lavender

This oil is perhaps the most versatile when it comes to healing. It exudes a sweet, flowery and fresh scent and is effective in treating the following:

- Stress and anxiety
- Depression
- High blood pressure
- Flatulence
- Whooping cough
- Panic attacks
- Bruises
- Oily skin
- Vertigo and earache
- Stretch marks

Peppermint

Aside from being a popular ingredient to freshen breath, peppermint is also useful as a natural remedy for the following:

- Gastrointestinal disorders
- Nasal congestion

- Headaches
- Lethargy
- Mental fatigue
- Asthma
- Nausea
- Pre-menstrual syndrome or PMS
- Itchiness
- Sore throat

Frankincense

Its aroma is a combination of sweet, fruity, woody and balsamic that stimulates cognitive functions. This essential oil can also deliver powerful results in the treatment of the following:

- Brain damage from injuries and trauma to the head
- Insecurity
- Grief
- Headaches
- Herpes
- Stress and anxiety
- Scars
- Bronchitis
- Allergies
- Strengthening the immune system

Cedar Wood

Extracted from Cedar Wood tree, this oil exudes a woody, sharp yet sweet scent. It is useful in treating the following:

- Seborrhoeic Eczema
- Psoriasis
- Tetanus
- Arthritis pain
- Spasm and spasmodic conditions

- Toothaches
- Diarrhea
- Obesity
- Urinary tract infection
- Gonorrhea

Sandalwood

From the oil of Sandalwood tree comes a distinct flora scent that is both sweet and rich. This oil is effective as a natural remedy for:

- Fertility and endocrine health
- Skin infections and disorders
- Gingivitis
- Scar healing
- Urinary tract infection
- Internal infections
- Viral infections such as cough and cold, flu, mumps
- Fever
- Hypertension
- Stress and anxiety

You may also want to check <u>Dr. Oz's Essential Oil Guide</u> for other oils that can treat ailments and conditions not mentioned in this chapter.

Chapter 6: How Oil Pulling Can Improve Your Oral Health

It pays to pay attention to your oral health. One of the most effective and yet the most affordable ways to improve your oral health is through oil pulling. In this chapter, you will learn about: (a) how to perform oil pulling; (b) what benefits you can get from doing it.

What is Oil Pulling

If you haven't heard about it yet, oil pulling is a traditional method of gargling using oil to "pull" dirt and bacteria and prevent the buildup of plague. Sesame oil, sunflower oil and coconut oil are three of the common oils used for this purpose.

How to Do It: What Oil to Use

Traditional experts recommend sesame or sunflower oil for this procedure. In recent studies, however, pure coconut oil appears to be the better choice because of the following:

- It contains antibacterial and antiviral properties proven to protect and promote oral health.

- Mixed with baking soda, you will be able to produce a natural teeth whitening toothpaste that also fights and prevents tooth decay.

- It can kill Candida Albicans that cause oral thrush.

Procedure

Follow these steps to benefit from oil pulling in promoting your oral health:

1. Choose the oil that you would like to use for oil pulling. As soon as you wake up in the morning, before putting anything into your mouth, take about two (2) tablespoons of your preferred oil. Swish and gargle the oil, but be careful not to swallow it. Do this for approximately 20 minutes.

2. Spit the oil, but not on your sink or toilet to prevent clogged pipes. After spitting the oil, proceed with your usual dental care routine, i.e. tooth brushing, flossing, and rinsing. Repeat step #1 and this step in the evening before you hit the sack.

What You Can Benefit from Oil Pulling

Scientific evidence points to how oil pulling can improve your oral health, as it can do the following:

- Get rid of dirt, impurities and other microbes residing in between your teeth, gums and mouth
- Prevent the accumulation of plague
- Remove and prevent bad odor in the mouth
- Treat and prevent bleeding gums
- Cure and prevent throat dryness
- Cure and prevent cracked lips
- Strengthen your teeth and gums

Oil pulling has benefits other than improving your oral health. These other benefits are still debatable. However, according to certain studies and testimonies from users, oil pulling can also detoxify the body and treat systemic diseases such as acne, cough and colds, and yeast infection to name some.

Why Oil Pulling is Beneficial

The reasons oil pulling is beneficial to your oral health are the following:

- It reduces the number of bacteria that cause tooth decay.
- It prevents plague build up and promotes gum health.
- It kills microorganisms that cause foul odor or bad breath.
- Evidence exists that oil pulling performs mechanical cleaning action in the mouth that stops and prevent oral diseases.

Chapter 7: How These Herbs & Spices Can Be Your Best Anti-Aging Natural Solution

Why spend your hard-earned money for anti aging products when you can get the same results from herbal remedies? In this chapter, you'll get to know five (5) of the best anti-aging herbs and spices you can use as your natural solution for the most common signs of aging.

Turmeric

Dr. Mehmet Oz, Dr. Joseph Mercola, and Dr. David Williams consider turmeric as one of the best spices to fight and delay not only the signs of aging, but also its effects on the health. Turmeric does not only inhibit the growth of cancer cells, but it can also prevent Alzheimer's disease.

Curcumin, the substance responsible for the yellow color of turmeric, is a potent antioxidant that protects the body against free radicals. It is also one of the most powerful anti-inflammatory spices that can shield the body and mind from degenerative diseases.

Marjoram

This aromatic herb belongs to the mint family and is the twin sibling of oregano. It delays the aging process by doing two crucial things: (1) promotes better sleep; and (2) improves digestion.

Marjoram is also a good stress reliever. You know how stress can make you look older than your age. This is because stress damages the cells that trigger the formation of frown lines, one of the signs of aging.

Ginseng

A popular Chinese herbal remedy, this plant is also a hit among the skin care population. This is because ginseng is effective in preserving youthful-looking skin by doing the following: delay the visible signs of aging such as wrinkles, prevent age spots and acne breakouts, restores youthful skin glow and gets rid of impurities and skin blemishes.

It is in the root of this plant where you can find concentrated phytonutrients that prevent aging and drying of the skin. These antioxidants also boost cell regeneration and repair damages of free radicals.

Bilberry

Wild blueberry or bilberry has the highest Oxygen Radical Absorbance Capacity (ORAC) among several fruits and berries. This berry is rich in resveratrol, vitamins E and C, ellagic acid, and anthocyanin, nutrients that benefit the skin.

What the nutrients in bilberry do is they neutralize enzymes that damage skin cells and connective tissues. This is what makes it effective in fighting the signs of skin aging such as sagging, wrinkles, age spots, and dryness among others.

Jamaican Pimento

This spice promotes heart health by maintaining the youthfulness of your arteries. It also helps regulate glucose or your blood sugar levels. It promotes healthy digestion so you can stay away from disorders and diseases that will speed up the aging process.

You simply have to add these herbs and spices to your meals to start benefiting from their anti-aging properties. These herbs and spices are rich in nutrients, thereby increasing the nutrient density of your meals. They also encourage you to drink more water, the best cleansing agent that can also be your fountain of youth.

Chapter 8: Discover The Medicinal Benefits Of Honey

From Mother Nature, you will find your best natural medicines. One of these is honey, which enjoys a long history of medicinal benefits. The ancient people used honey to treat, disinfect and heal wounds. Today, honey remains to be one of the best ways to treat and cure wounds.

Wound Care

The best proof of the medicinal properties of honey comes from its ability to treat and heal wounds. Countless of studies confirm the effectiveness of honey in the treatment of wounds even those that are extremely difficult to heal.

This is because of the following:

- Anti-microbial action - As soon as honey touches the wound, the contact allows for the production of hydrogen peroxide that works gradually to kill microbes without damaging skin tissues.

- Phytochemicals – Especially with Manuka honey, the rich amount of phytochemicals present in the substance enables the restoration of skin cells for faster wound healing.

- Phagocytes – Honey enhances the functions of the white blood cells (phagocytes), thereby shielding the body systems from infectious microorganisms. These cells also improve the immune response of the body against harmful microbes.

Antibacterial

According to experts at the WebMD, honey inhibits the growth of food-borne microorganisms, e.g. Salmonella and E. coli. It is also effective in eliminating bacteria, e.g. Staphylococcus aureus as well as Pseudomonas aeruginosa. These bacteria can cause a range of diseases from skin infections to life-threatening ailments such as acne and abscess to meningitis and sepsis.

Weight Loss

If you wish to lose weight more effectively, you can count on one ingredient to do its job well. That ingredient is honey. While honey contains more calories compared to sugar, when you add it to warm water or to lemon or to both, it acts as a fat burner.

Honey contains nutrients that can lower your high blood cholesterol and regulate your high blood sugar. To maximize your weight loss benefits, combine honey with any or all of the following: warm water, lemon and cinnamon.

Honey Weight Loss Recipe

Here's a quick weight loss recipe using honey as an ingredient:

Ingredients	1 tablespoon of raw honey 1 teaspoon of organic cinnamon 1 cup of purified water
Procedure	1. Boil the purified water. 2. Place your cinnamon in a bowl. Pour the boiled water over it and steep for about 15 minutes or until the water is just warm. 3. Add the honey to the warm water with cinnamon.

	Tip: Avoid adding honey to hot or boiling water since the heat usually destroys enzymes and nutrients present in it. Cool the water first until it's warm before adding honey for weight loss.

Benefits You Can Enjoy from the Recipe

The honey in the recipe works as a speedy fat burner, while at the same time preventing blood sugar spikes. Cinnamon, for its part, increases the efficiency of blood sugar metabolism that prevents unnecessary storage of fats in the body.

Both honey and cinnamon will allow you to feel fuller longer, so you will be able to control your appetite and to get rid of your food cravings. Aside from the weight loss benefits, this recipe also gives you more energy and improves your sexual drive.

Chapter 9: How To Use Apple Cider Vinegar For Weight Loss

Aside from honey, apple cider vinegar proves to deliver guaranteed weight loss results without adverse effects. The best thing about using apple cider vinegar for weight loss is that it can detoxify your body to optimize the functions of your body systems. This chapter focuses on how you can use apple cider vinegar or ACV to deliver proven weight loss results.

ACV Natural Weight Loss Formula

The formula to lose weight with apple cider vinegar is extremely simple:

Weight loss = 2 tablespoons of ACV + 16 oz. of water

With this formula, you can create your weight loss solution easily. All you need to do is to drink the ACV water at least once daily or up to three times daily before taking your meal(s). If you choose to take it once a day, the best time to drink your ACV water is right after you wake up in the morning or before taking your breakfast.

How to Start Benefiting from ACV Water

If you are just starting to benefit from ACV water in terms of losing your excess weight, begin with a modified formula, as follows:

Initial Weight Loss – 1 teaspoon of ACV + 16 oz. of water

Drink your ACV water once daily, preferably before breakfast, until you acquire the taste. Slowly increase the amount of apple cider vinegar until you reach and are able to follow the standard formula. Do the same for the frequency of drinking your ACV water solution. Start with once a day until you reach the maximum of three times a day.

If, however, despite your determination and effort to acquire the taste, you find it difficult to drink your ACV water, what you can do is to add a few drops of honey (preferably organic or raw honey) to make it more palatable.

How ACV Water Works to Get Rid of Excess Weight

Apple cider vinegar contains acids and enzymes that boost metabolism and activate the body's natural fat burning mechanism. Its natural chemicals eliminate toxic substances that interfere with your body systems resulting to unnecessary fat storage.

The acid and enzymes work together to normalize your blood sugar, preventing spikes or sudden rush. Regulated blood sugar is essential to help the body get rid of its unnecessary fats. Additionally, apple cider vinegar restores the alkalinity your body needs to maintain its good health condition.

Sample ACV Weight Loss Recipe

Here is a sample recipe to benefit from apple cider vinegar for weight loss:

Ingredients	2 tablespoons of apple cider vinegar (adjust accordingly) 1 teaspoon of raw honey 16 oz. distilled or purified lukewarm water (you may increase the amount of water)
Procedure	1. In a bottle, pour your lukewarm water and then add your apple cider vinegar. Shake well. 2. Add the honey and then shake

	the solution well.
	Tip: Similar to honey, never add apple cider vinegar to hot or boiling water as the heat will only destroy its enzymes and nutrients. Allow the water to cool until it's warm or lukewarm.

Aside from this recipe, you can also use apple cider vinegar in recipes requiring you to use vinegar as an ingredient. Substituting your regular vinegar with ACV can transform the recipe and produce healthier meals for weight loss.

Chapter 10: Sustainable Gardening Of Herbal Plants

In this chapter, you will learn the basics of sustainable gardening so that you can grow herbs you can use to create your own natural remedies.

Best Herbs to Grow for Beginners

Here are the three (3) best herbal plants to grow if you are just beginning your garden of herbs:

1. Basil – Choose the sweet variety because aside from having more fragrance and flavor, it is also the fastest-growing plant. To start growing, plant your basil in your garden plot or container filled with <u>organic nutrients</u>. Make sure that your plant receives enough sunlight, as basil loves warm environment to grow well.

2. Mint – requires minimal supervision that makes it suitable for those who are just starting to grow their herbal garden. The best way to plant this herb is to place it in bottomless pot before replanting it in the soil where it can receive sunlight. Fill the soil with organic nutrients and watch how your mint grows fast.

3. Parsley – grows well in nutrient-rich soil in full sun or partial shade. It requires minimal care like the basil and mint, but parsley may take a little longer time to grow (if you grow it from seeds). After seed germination, the plant will grow rapidly and easily. Start growing it, therefore, from transplants.

Basic Rules

Follow these basic rules in sustainable gardening:

- Choose a place where your herbal plants can receive adequate sunlight and where you can easily and conveniently water your plants.

- Soil has to be nutrient-rich and free from impurities such as weeds, rocks, rubbish and others that can hamper the growth of your plants.

- Choose the right time to plant. Some herbs grow best under full sun, while others can do well even with partial shade.

- Make sure to remove weeds that may grow with your plants. These weeds will compete with your plants for the nutrients in the soil.

- Never allow your plants to dry by watering them to preserve soil moisture. Avoid the temptation to excessively water your plants, as this may drown them.

- Harvest your herbal plants only when they are mature. This way, you can enjoy their best appearance, flavor, aroma and health benefits.

Even in compact spaces, you can still start your sustainable herbal garden. The best part of growing your plants is that you will be able to enjoy organic herbs free from pesticides and other harmful chemicals typical to commercially grown ones.

Conclusion

Thank you again for purchasing this book on *"Incredible Herbal Remedies! - Herbs, Spices, And Oils To Cure Common Ailments, Prevent Sickness, Improve Health And Fight Disease!"*

I am extremely excited to pass this information along to you, and I am so happy that you now have read and can hopefully implement these strategies going forward.

I hope this book was able to help you understand the potentials and power of using natural remedies

- To treat common ailments and diseases,
- To delay the aging process, shield the body against the effects of aging, and to maintain youthful-looking skin;
- To improve overall health condition; as well as
- How you can grow your own herbal garden sustainably.

Using herbal remedies has several benefits and in many instances, these are more advantageous than depending on drug-based medicines. What this book suggests is to minimize your use of pharmaceuticals and start benefiting from herbs, spices, and essential oils.

It is also best that you maintain your consultation with your physician and discuss how you can integrate the use of herbal remedies to fight ailments and prevent diseases. The best physician is open to exploring all possible solutions to improve health and to treat conditions using natural remedies, especially those that do not require immediate medical intervention.

The next step is to get started using this information and to hopefully live a healthier life without having to use and spend much for drug-based medications and treatments unless they are necessary.

Please don't be someone who just reads this information and doesn't apply it, the strategies in this book will only benefit you if you use them!

If you know of anyone else that could benefit from the information presented here please inform them of this book.

Finally, if you enjoyed this book and feel it has added value to your life in any way, please take the time to share your thoughts and post a review on Amazon. It'd be greatly appreciated!

Thank you and good luck!

Preview Of:

Ancient Natural Beauty Secrets!

Natural Beauty

Organic Superfoods, Essential Oils, Natural Remedies, Homemade Beauty Recipes, Skin Care Secrets, And More Tips For Anti Aging And Youthful Appearance!

Introduction

I want to thank you and congratulate you for purchasing the book, *"Ancient Natural Beauty Secrets! Organic Superfoods, Essential Oils, Natural Remedies, Homemade Beauty Recipes, Skin Care Secrets, And More Tips For Anti Aging And Youthful Appearance!"*

This book contains proven steps and strategies on how to stay youthful through the years with the use of ancient but effective natural beauty remedies. This book also teaches you the essentials in staying beautiful and glowing through simple steps that you can do at home without spending a dime. This is a must-read for people who are aspiring to maintain their good looks in practical, risk-free and natural ways.

Thanks again for purchasing this book; I hope you enjoy it!

Chapter 1: Ancient Natural Beauty Secrets – What Are They?

Beauty concerns are universal. They've been and will remain an issue for the human race regardless of any age, gender or era. Can you imagine how people in the past managed to survive these beauty dilemmas?

People who lived in the ancient times have found their own ways to achieve ageless beauty. They were curious, driven and brave enough to experiment with their only resource – nature. Luckily for mankind, nature has all the answers. Take a sneak peek at these ancient beauty secrets!

Beauty tips and tricks come and go; they rise and fall according to the latest beauty trends. However, there are some beauty secrets which stood the test of time. These classic beauty secrets have proven themselves to be more resilient than a beauty hype that everybody forgets after a week and that is simply because they deliver on their promises consistently.

But what's so good about these ancient beauty secrets that would get you dying to try and stick to them for good? Here are some of them:

Ancient beauty solutions are natural

Going back to the past might be helpful when it comes to beauty ideas. The pureness of the materials they use back then (when there was nothing but nature to turn to) is simply too good to forget. There were no harmful chemicals to speak of, only pure natural goodness.

Ancient beauty solutions are raw

Our elders did not care much about product processing. Without the technological breakthroughs during that time, you cannot really expect their beauty products to be as carefully processed as the products sold in the market today. This would only mean one thing – ancient beauty remedies are made from nothing less than raw and roughly processed materials in its purest and most natural state. As such, it retains most of the natural goodness that it contains which would otherwise be stripped off by product processing.

Ancient beauty solutions do not trigger harmful effects

These ancient secrets are made of pure natural goodness which causes little or no harm at all to the body. This would mean fewer health concerns and worry about the things you're putting in your body. By using natural beauty remedies, you can always have the peace of mind knowing that you can get beautiful without compromising your health.

Ancient beauty solutions are usually cheap and even FREE!

Ancient beauty treats are all good news for anyone who wants to get beautiful on a budget. The good thing about these ancient beauty items is that most of them can be found in your backyard or kitchen. They don't always have to be in an expensive salon or spa that you can't afford to go to every single time a pimple or two pops out. All of these lead us to believe in one thing: *you can never put a price on beauty!*

Thanks for Previewing My Exciting Book Entitled:

"Natural Beauty: Ancient Natural Beauty Secrets! Organic Superfoods, Essential Oils, Natural Remedies, Homemade Beauty Recipes, Skin Care Secrets, And More Tips For Anti Aging And Youthful Appearance!"

To purchase this book, simply go to the Amazon Kindle store and simply search:

"NATURAL BEAUTY"

Then just scroll down until you see my book. You will know it is mine because you will see my name "Sarah Brooks" underneath the title.

Alternatively, you can visit my author page on Amazon to see this book and other work I have done. Thanks so much, and please don't forget your free bonuses

DON'T LEAVE YET! - CHECK OUT YOUR FREE BONUSES BELOW!

Free Bonus Offer: Get Free Access To The www.LuxyLifeNaturals.com VIP Newsletter!

Once you enter your email address you will immediately get free access to this awesome newsletter!

But wait, right now if you join now for free you will also get free access the "Secrets of Becoming A Meditation Expert – In 7 Days!" free Ebook!

To claim both your FREE VIP NEWSLETTER MEMBERSHIP and your FREE BONUS Ebook on the SECRETS OF BECOMING A MEDITATION EXPERT IN 7 DAYS!

Just Go To:

www.LuxyLifeNaturals.com